I0428939

45 DAYS TO BADASS:
FITNESS MOTIVATION

BY
JULIA PRESS SIMMONS

Published by Julia Press Simmons
Copyright © 2016 by Julia Press Simmons

All rights reserved. Without limiting the rights under copyright reserved above. No part of this book may be reproduced, stored in or introduced into a retrieval system, or transmitted in any form, or by any means (electronic, mechanical, photocopying, recording, or otherwise), without prior written consent from the author, except brief quotes used in reviews.

ISBN-13:
978-1530027569

ISBN-10:
153002756X

www.JPSimmons.ninja
www.instagram.com/bravegirlology
www.twitter.com/jpsimmons
www.facbook.com/JPSBOOKS

<u>Disclaimer</u>

These ideas and suggestions written by Julia Press Simmons are provided as general educational information only. It should not be construed as medical advice or care. All matters regarding your health require supervision by a personal physician or other appropriate healthcare professionals familiar with your current health status. Always consult a personal physician before making any dietary or exercise changes. Julia Press Simmons and Royalty Press disclaim any liability or warranties of any kind arriving directly or indirectly from the use of this information if any medical problems develop always consult your personal physician. Only your physician can provide you with medical advice. Throughout this document or links to external sites. These external sites contain information created and maintained by other individuals in organizations and are provided for the user's convenience Julia Press-Simmons and royalty price do not control nor can they guarantee the accuracy, relevance, timeliness , or completeness of this information neither is it intended to endorse any view or express its importance by including it in this book.

<u>ACKNOWLEDGEMENTS</u>

I would like to thank my family for the love, laughter, and inspiration. I promise to always write my heart out for all of you!

Motivation will almost always beat mere talent.
-Norman R. Augustine

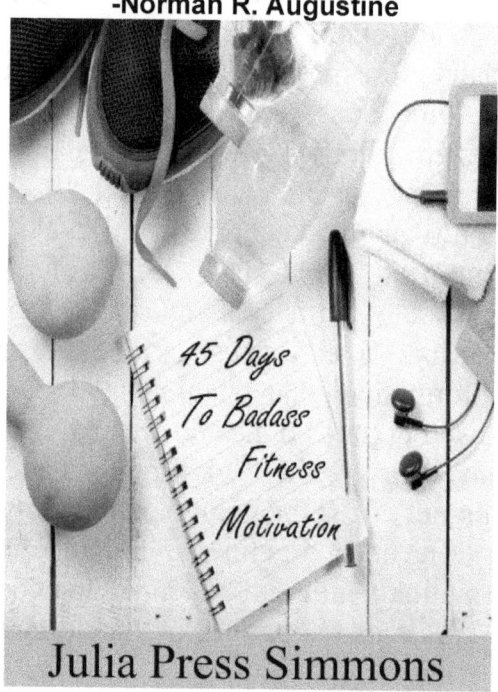

Julia Press Simmons

45 Days to Badass is designed to offer daily motivation for anyone on a weight loss journey. It is

full of my favorite quotes, video links, and personal triumphs.
"People often say that motivation doesn't last. Well, neither does bathing, that's why we recommend it daily." Zig Ziglar

FOR DAILY MOTIVATION SIGN UP FOR MY FREE NEWSLETTER

HERE

INTRODUCTION

"Motivation is what gets you started. Habit is what keeps you going."--Jim Ryan

Dear Readers/family,

There will be three major themes and several minor themes repeated throughout this book. The repetition is deliberate, and similar to how we are given information throughout our learning lives. It is my intention that the book's message not only hits home for you, but it becomes second nature and that you practice these things long after you read the last line on the last page.

With Love & Sincerity
Julia Press Simmons

THREE MAJOR THEMES

MOTIVATION ~ Defined as the reason or reasons one has for acting or behaving in a particular way. The general desire or willingness of someone to do something.

DETERMINATION ~ Defined as firmness of purpose. Resoluteness. The process of establishing something exactly, typically by calculation or research.

FOCUS ~ Defined as the center of interest or activity. The state or quality of having or producing clear visual definition. To pay particular attention to.

HOW TO USE THIS BOOK

45 Days to Badass is designed to deliver daily motivation and support to anyone looking to achieve a healthier lifestyle. You could sit back with a nice cup of herbal tea and read this book cover to cover, but that would defeat the purpose. For the next 45 days you should wake up, read the corresponding page, meditate on the message, watch the YouTube motivational video, and complete the assignment. This book is a contract with yourself. It is a commitment to make yourself a priority.

EVERY PRO WAS
ONCE AN AMATEUR.
EVERY EXPERT WAS
ONCE A BEGINNER.
SO DREAM BIG.
AND START NOW.

DAY ONE

The secret of getting ahead is getting started.
-Mark Twain

MEDITATION~ I will value myself enough to give 100% every time.

SUGGESTED VIDEO~ https://youtu.be/hbnrb0BMBtQ

You have already won. You're a certified winner, a fucking superstar. You've decided to take control over your life; mind, body and spirit. You've decided to make yourself a priority, and you feel amazing about the decision. Today you've declared in a loud voice, "I AM WORTH MY BEST EFFORT, AND I AM GOING TO PROVE IT." Awesome! Today is the first day of badassery, and your assignment is simple...

1. 15 to 30 minutes of exercise
2. drink 8 glasses of water
3. write down your goals and objectives for the day/week/month

DAY 1 NOTES

DAY TWO

"Don't let the fear of losing be greater than the excitement of winning."--Robert Kiyosaki

MEDITATION~ I will be positive in all things. I choose to see the good in every situation.

SUGGESTED VIDEO~ https://youtu.be/NMDw-PxA828

The battle for health and wellness begins and ends in your mind. It is imperative that you keep a positive outlook on fitness. Exercise is hard and demanding, but it's not the physical aspect of the activity that stops you, it's your perception of it. A positive attitude will make your journey amazing. The simple mental switch of looking at fitness as a plus can change everything... You don't have to work out, you get to work out. Every time you have a negative thought combat it with a positive one. Second day of badassery assignment is as follows.

1. 15 to 30 minutes of exercise
2. drink eight glasses of water
3. list 10 positive reasons why fitness is important

DAY 2 NOTES

DAY THREE

"All our dreams can come true if we have the courage to pursue them."--Walt Disney

MEDITATION~ I am disciplined and dedicated to achieving my goals.

SUGGESTED VIDEO~ https://youtu.be/hbnrb0BMBtQ

It takes courage to change your life. You can't be a weak willed little bitch, and expect to see results. Life doesn't work that way. "Fortune favors the bold." You must be fierce to achieve your goals. The good thing about courage is that we all have it, every human on the planet is born with it. Just like fear is taught and reinforced by society, you can learn to be brave. As you embark on this health and wellness journey you will feel the fear of failure. It can paralyze you if you let it, but you are not about to let it. You will feel the fear, but press on anyway. This is how you become bold. This is how you become brave. Today's badassery assignment is as follows.

1. 15 to 30 minutes of exercise
2. drink 8 glasses of water
3. write down 3 of your biggest fitness fears, and then demolish them.

DAY 3 NOTES

DAY FOUR

"I find that the harder I work, the more luck I seem to have."--Thomas Jefferson

MEDITATION~ With each passing day I gain more control over my impulses.

SUGGESTED VIDEO~ https://youtu.be/8EGWEUf9Xr8

Everywhere you look from social media and broadcast television; to the magazines in the checkout line at your neighborhood grocery store you can find a get slim quick scheme. They all offer the virtual magic pill that will get you to your desired weight, fitness level, and overall state of wellness with little to no effort on your part. That, my friend, is a lie. Changing your lifestyle, mindset, and physical wellbeing is a mighty effort that requires daily doses of hard work. The grind needed to obtain all of your goals isn't a bad thing. It's beautiful. Hard work is transformative, uplifting, and its results are undeniable. You can't cheat the grind it knows how much effort you put in, and it shows it to the world.

1. 15 to 30 minutes of exercise
2. Drink 8 glasses of water
3. List 3 hard things that are stopping you from achieving your goals. Then list 3 ways to overcome them. Hard work should never be a deterrent.

DAY 4 NOTES

_____

_____

_____

_____

_____

_____

_____

_____

_____

_____

_____

_____

_____

_____

DAY FIVE

"To accomplish great things, we must not only act, but also dream, not only plan, but also believe."--Anatole France

MEDITATION~ I am only influenced by positive beliefs and thoughts.

SUGGESTED VIDEO~ https://youtu.be/OMDXTeqGo3A

I cannot stress how important it is to believe in yourself. Have faith in abilities. Tell yourself that you are strong and capable of great things. Tell yourself that you are worth of your very best and believe those statements with everything that's in you. When I look back on my life, all of my failures and all of my accomplishments were the direct effect of my mindset. "If you think you can, or if you think you can't you are right. I personally believe that you are capable of greatness. I need for you to believe it to. Fifth day of badassery assignment is as follows.

1. 15 to 30 minutes of exercise
2. Drink 8 glasses of water
3. List 5 things you would do if you believed you wouldn't fail.

DAY 5 NOTES

DAY SIX

"The successful warrior is the average man, with laser-like focus."--Bruce Lee

MEDITATION~ I am free from distractions I stay focused on the task at hand.

SUGGESTED VIDEO~ https://youtu.be/hqAKw9aZu1E

You can overcome any and all adversity with focused deliberate action if you are persistent you can achieve anything you want. If you are consistent you can keep the success you worked so hard for. Every day you will encounter distractions life doesn't stop being a bitch because you chose to adopt a healthy lifestyle. When your days become long and hard you will need to remain focused on your goals. Whenever I'd go through emotional, physical, or mental stress I would overeat and use food and sloth to soothe myself. And, all of my fitness and weight loss goals went out the window. I learned to stop hurting myself when I'm hurting and to focus on my goals throughout life's trials. Sixth Day of badassery assignment is as follows;

1. 15 to 30 minutes of exercise
2. Drink 8 glasses of water
3. List 3 major distractions in your life and plan to reduce them by 50%

DAY 6 NOTES

DAY SEVEN

"The last three or four reps is what makes the muscle grow. This area of pain divides the champion from someone else who is not a champion." - *Schwarzenegger*

MEDITATION~ Every day I am more determined than ever to realize my goals.

SUGGESTED VIDEO~ https://youtu.be/l_Yg6F7OOQE

Congratulations you made it through the first week of your new way of life. You did the hard work. You made yourself a priority. You believed in yourself, and you remained focus. I wish I could tell you that it gets easier from here on out, but this book is not fiction. Changing your life is no easy day at the beach. This isn't light work, this will not get easier but if you remain determined to achieve your goal you will get stronger. The seventh day of badassery assignment is as follows;

1. 15 to 30 minutes of exercise
2. Drink 8 glasses of water
3. List 5 things you find hard about working out, and then list how you overcome them.

DAY 7 NOTES

DAY EIGHT

"There's no secret formula. I lift heavy, work hard, and aim to be the best."

- Ronnie Coleman, eight-time Mr. Olympia

MEDITATION~ I am successful in every aspect of my life. In everyday in every way, I get better and better.

SUGGESTED VIDEO~ https://youtu.be/BW3EA0AdZx0

I can't lie, crunches hurt LIKE HELL, burpees are from the devil, and Russian twist makes you hate life. However if you want the extra minutes off of your hourglass figure you have to do that shit, and trust me eventually you will learn to love it. There is sweet satisfaction that comes from mastering an exercise that you didn't think you would ever be able to do. On top of the endorphins your body will reward you with from the physical activity; you will gain a sense of pride and confidence that will seep into other areas of your life. The eighth day of badassery assignment is as follows;

1. 15 to 30 minutes of exercise
2. Drink 8 glasses of water
3. List 3 exercises that you find hard to do, and then make a promise to yourself to conquer them.

DAY 8 NOTES

DAY NINE

Strive for progress, not perfection.
-Unknown

MEDITATION~ every day I take at least one positive step towards my goal, and every day I get a little closer.

SUGGESTED VIDEO~ https://youtu.be/xmPuzWRIVJw

Perfection is a myth. There is no perfect weight, size, or figure. Many people fail at their weight loss goals because the chase something unobtainable. They draw hard lines in the sand and get discouraged when a strong wind sweeps in and blows the line away. They adopt a diet mentality, instead of embracing a lifestyle change. Then they tell themselves that they will be a certain weight or size by a certain date and fall into despair when they don't hit their marks. This is foolish. Arthur Ashe said it best, "start where you are, use what you have, and do what you can." Focus on improving every day, and the results will take care of themselves. The ninth day of badassery assignment is as follows;

1. 15 to 30 minutes of exercise
2. Drink 8 glasses of water
3. List 3 long term lifestyle goals.

DAY 9 NOTES

DAY TEN

If you don't make mistakes, you aren't really trying.
-Unknown

MEDITATION~ I accept myself even though I make mistakes. I am worth my kindness and my forgiveness

SUGGESTED VIDEO~ https://youtu.be/mgmVOuLgFB0

You had a double cheeseburger with bacon and all the extras. You drank a big ass margarita and then had a couple bowls of ice cream. You skipped a workout and then another one. You are starting to feel like shit, like all hope is lost, but this is just a feeling. It is not the end of the world. Mistakes are human nature. It happens, and since this is a journey and not a diet you get up off your ass, dust yourself off and fight another day. Don't let a mistake mess with the mission. Ain't, nobody got time for that. Fall down seven times stand up eight. Remember a time that you fucked up royally and realize you didn't die. The tenth day of badassery assignment is as follows;

1. 15 to 30 minutes of exercise
2. Drink 8 glasses of water
3. List 3 mistakes you made in life, and then the outcome of those mistakes. Search for the lesson

DAY 10 NOTES

DAY ELEVEN

**Ability is what you're capable of doing.
Motivation determines what you do. Attitude
determines how well you do it.
-Lou Holtz**

MEDITATION~ I am responsible for my own beliefs
and attitudes.

SUGGESTED VIDEO~ https://youtu.be/Eu_dUxTg33l

"Your attitude determines your altitude" I
remember reading that quote on my guidance
counselor's wall in high school. She would point to
it when my attitude got a little funky, and then she
would remind me that I would never get anywhere
in life until I changed it. Change that attitude
people would say, but they never really told me
how. I learned the hard way, but I learned.
Gratefulness is the most powerful attitude changer.
If you are thankful and constantly counting your
blessings, it is near impossible to have a negative
outlook on life. Once you have a positive outlook
the path ahead become clear, and your goals
suddenly appear in arms reach. The tenth day of
badassery assignment is as follows;

1. 15 to 30 minutes of exercise
2. Drink 8 glasses of water
3. List 10 blessings in your life

DAY 11 NOTES

DAY TWELVE

Strength does not come from physical capacity. It comes from an indomitable will.
-Mahatma Gandhi

MEDITATION~ My body is healthy; my mind is brilliant; my soul is tranquil.

SUGGESTED VIDEO~ https://youtu.be/RXI6QpWQ5xo

Your will power is a muscle and like all muscles it can be strengthened with repetitive training. Every Time you exert your will you make it stronger saying no to being lazy and unproductive strengthen you will. Choosing the salad over the cheeseburger strengthen your will. Positive choices and decisions strengthens your will, and the stronger you will becomes, the more control you gain over your life and its directions. The twelfth day of badassery assignment is as follows;

1. 15 to 30 minutes of exercise
2. Drink 8 glasses of water
3. List 3 unhealthy habits that you will defeat today.

DAY 12 NOTES

DAY THIRTEEN

It's not who you are that holds you back, it's who you think you're not.
-Anonymous

MEDITATION~ Today, I abandon my old habits and take up new, more positive ones.

SUGGESTED VIDEO~ https://youtu.be/yecahBzZwqo

Self-confidence is defined as a feeling of self-assurance arising from one's appreciation of one's own abilities and qualities. Failure to achieve your dream is rooted in the fact that you don't believe can achieve it, or worse yet you don't really believe that you deserve it. That is a big ol' red light in your life. You are stopping yourself from obtaining your heart's desire because you don't love yourself enough. You don't think you are worthy, and that should stop today. You deserve it all. You are beautiful expression of love and life and you should treat yourself accordingly. The thirteenth day of badassery assignment is as follows;

1. 15 to 30 minutes of exercise
2. Drink 8 glasses of water
3. List 5 things that you love about yourself

DAY 13 NOTES

DAY FOURTEEN

Clear your mind of can't.
-Samuel Johnson

MEDITATION~ I deserve all that is good. I release any need for misery and suffering.

SUGGESTED VIDEO~ https://youtu.be/aDCGrINPGUQ

Congratulations you made to week 2 and it's about time you eliminate the word can't from your vocabulary. Every single reason you have of why you can't do something is an excuse, and excuses are for pussies, and I'm no vagina. I have one but I'm not one. The day I let go of can't was the most powerful day of my life. A world of possibilities was suddenly available to me. I realized that the "I CAN" and "I WILL" mindset is the keys to freedom. Let go of can't replace it with I can. You are the architect of your life. You are the designer and you are in control you can do anything you want to do in this life. BELIEVE!!! The fourteenth day of badassery assignment is as follows;

1. 15 to 30 minutes of exercise
2. Drink 8 glasses of water
3. List 3 things that you think you can't do, and do them!

DAY 14 NOTES

DAY FIFTEEN

"You must expect great things in your life before you can do them."--Michael Jordan

MEDITATION~ I visualize positive change and manifest it into reality

SUGGESTED VIDEO~ https://youtu.be/d4h7pbn8pF4

Take a moment and visualize the life you want. Where are you physically? How is your health? Are you spiritually connected? Are you emotionally stable? Are you financially secure? The first step to obtaining any goal is visualization. Your imagination is a powerful tool that is sadly underused when we become adults. I have a vision of the women I want to be, in my head, and I work towards that vision every day. At first it seemed silly and the body I imagined seemed like a fantasy, but I remained faithful to my dream, and worked my ass off 6 days a week. The pounds started melting off and the woman I imagined started to appear. The fifteenth day of badassery assignment is as follows;

4. 15 to 30 minutes of exercise
5. Drink 8 glasses of water
6. List 5 things that you visualize changing about yourself

DAY 15 NOTES

DAY SIXTEEN

Energy and persistence conquer all things.
-Benjamin Franklin

MEDITATION~ I am a powerhouse; I am indestructible.

SUGGESTED VIDEO~ https://youtu.be/_pi7oqZ6ioU

The power of persistence is awesome. You can climb a mountain. You can swim an ocean. You can walk across the country with persistence. Any adversity can be overcome with relentless action. The first leg of your journey to fitness can be uneventful. When I started to exercise I would go hard for days and days with little to no results. The scale didn't move, my clothes were not falling off and I started to get discouraged. I almost gave up. But, I was so tired of giving up. I knew that nothing would change if I stopped, so I didn't quit. I kept at it. I stopped getting on the scale constantly. I purchased new clothes that made me feel beautiful and sexy at my current size. And, above all, I kept going and now my persistence is starting to pay off. The sixteenth day of badassery assignment is as follows;

1. 15 to 30 minutes of exercise
2. Drink 8 glasses of water
3. List 3 small changes that you can make everyday

DAY 16 NOTES

DAY SEVENTEEN

"If it doesn't challenge you, it doesn't change you."
Fred Devito

MEDITATION~ I have more than enough strength and vigor to complete my goals.

SUGGESTED VIDEO~ https://youtu.be/CMm6tDavSXg

Losing weight, changing your lifestyle, and improving yourself and your outlook on life is difficult. It is meticulous and grueling. You will have road blocks. You will reach seemingly unbreakable plateaus. Life will knock you down and kick dirt in your face when you try to get up. Friends will abandon you. Family will belittle you. You will feel weak. It will all seem pointless. You'll want to give up 5, 10, 15 times a day, but you must keep going. You must develop the testicular fortitude to fight negativity and win. You are being forged in the fire. You are being transformed. If it was easy you would have done it a long time ago. The seventeenth day of badassery assignment is as follows;

1. 15 to 30 minutes of exercise
2. Drink 8 glasses of water
3. List 3 things that used to stop you in the past, and then list how you are going to overcome them.

DAY 17 NOTES

DAY EIGHTEEN

**"If you don't do what's best for your body,
you're the one who comes up on the short end."
~ Julius Erving**

MEDITATION~ I have the power to change myself

SUGGESTED VIDEO~ https://youtu.be/Vr7ysfZVXHE

Your meditation, your daily inspiration, your meal plan and your fitness routine is a beautiful expression of self-love. It is how you take care of yourself and it's important it is a vital component to the life you want and the life you deserve. Make your fitness routine a priority. Make it paramount then sit back and watch your life change in ways you never envisioned. The concept of self-love in regards to fitness is not expressed enough. You do not pushing your body to the limit at the gym or at home with various routines because you hate the way you look. It should be done because you love yourself so much that you will always do what is needed for you to obtain and maintain optimal health. The eighteenth day of badassery assignment is as follows;

4. 15 to 30 minutes of exercise
5. Drink 8 glasses of water
6. List 5 things you love about you

DAY 18 NOTES

DAY NINETEEN

"To keep the body in good health is a duty... otherwise we shall not be able to keep our mind strong and clear." ~ Buddha

MEDITATION~ I am free to choose to live as I wish and to give priority to my desires

SUGGESTED VIDEO~ https://youtu.be/Ps4hAQ_Fp5k

As hard as you're working, as much as you are sweating, as long as it took you to get to this stage of your journey, why would you sabotage yourself in any way? You don't feed your family poison. You don't cause them bodily harm or intentionally give them mental and emotional stress. So why would you do that to yourself? Respect your temple. Protect you from you. Your body needs water, so drink it, your heart needs cardio to remain strong so you must exercise, and your spirit requires peace and balance so you must pray and meditate. These things are not optional and shouldn't be treated as such. The nineteenth day of badassery assignment is as follows;

1. 15 to 30 minutes of exercise
2. Drink 8 glasses of water
3. List 5 nice things you do for others, and vow to be nicer to you!

DAY 19 NOTES

DAY TWENTY

"Those who think they have not time for bodily exercise will sooner or later have to find time for illness." ~ Edward Stanley

MEDITATION~ I am conquering my illness; I am defeating it steadily each day.

SUGGESTED VIDEO~ https://youtu.be/3GZxVAJBtg4

I beat diabetes, I reversed Type II Diabetes. In 2005 I weighed 275 lbs. and was diagnosed with type 2 diabetes. My father was an insulin dependent diabetic, so I was familiar with the disease, and It's devastating side effects. When I was diagnosed I slipped into a dark depression that I hid from my friends and family. My food addiction went into overdrive and in a few short years I ballooned up to 310 lbs. My father passed away from cancer in 2013 and that loss made me look at food and exercise in a different light. I started to change my thinking and reversed my diabetes with healthier food choices and exercise. The amount of diseases you can avoid or cure completely with a healthy lifestyle is staggering. No drugs, no doctors and no hospital bills. Just move your ass and eat right. Point, blank, and period. The twentieth day of badassery assignment is as follows;

1. 15 to 30 minutes of exercise
2. Drink 8 glasses of water
3. List all the things that negatively affect your health, and what you plan to do about it

DAY 20 NOTES

DAY TWENTY-ONE

"My temptation is emotional, and resisting will further my needed weight loss and strengthen my character. Furthermore, nothing tastes as good as thin feels." ~ Stephen Covey

MEDITATION~ Every day in every way I am approaching my ideal weight.

SUGGESTED VIDEO~ https://youtu.be/bfG0jgwDdSI

Week three and time for more visualization, so close your eyes and visualize your perfect body. What size are you? How much do you weigh? How do you feel? What style of clothes are your wearing? How is your hairstyle? Once you formed your ideal image of yourself commit every detailed memory and then start working towards it. Study it push yourself until you achieve it. Tell yourself that you can do it. Every morning and every night you are three weeks into your new way of life. Your dreams are within your reach all you have to do is keep striving and that vision will become a reality. The twenty-first day of badassery assignment is as follows;

1. 15 to 30 minutes of exercise
2. Drink 8 glasses of water
3. List 3 characteristics you want to acquire and what you plan to do to get them.

DAY 21 NOTES

DAY TWENTY-TWO

"If a man achieves victory over this body, who in the world can exercise power over him? He who rules himself rules over the whole world." – Vinoba Bhave

MEDITATION~ I am strong against negative life circumstances

SUGGESTED VIDEO~
https://youtu.be/oaxmq77kMVQ

When you commit to an exercise program, it causes a positive domino effect in your life. The discipline needed to workout everyday will spill over to everyday decisions. Your energy level is high, so you will find that you complete task easier. Your focus is sharper and your confidence is at an all-time high. Your self-discipline, self-esteem, and self-control have increased. You start to believe that you are capable of completing more tasks because you now have a proven track record of getting shit done. The decision to commit to a regular exercise routine cultivates discipline and discipline opens doors in your life that you didn't even know were closed. The twenty-second day of badassery assignment is as follows;

1. 15 to 30 minutes of exercise
2. Drink 8 glasses of water
3. List 3 new commitments

DAY 22 NOTES

DAY TWENTY-THREE

"Exercise equals endorphins. Endorphins makes you happy." **Unknown**

MEDITATION~ I can choose happiness whenever I wish no matter what my circumstances

SUGGESTED VIDEO~
https://youtu.be/QeGmdG0nnf4

The keys to happiness can be found at the end of every workout. It doesn't matter if it is in the gym or your living room, if you crush your workout you will be overjoyed. Happiness is a physiological reward gifted to you by your body for working out as hard as you can. That's not a Whistling Dixie I'm not pulling your leg. This is a fact, this is science. Exercise releases endorphins and endorphins are the happy hormone. They relieve stress, kill pain and are the key components of organisms. You read that right. Working out hard can have the same effect on your body as a sexual climax. If that ain't enough reason to give your workout your all, I don't know what is. The twenty-third day of badassery assignment is as follows;

1. 15 to 30 minutes of exercise
2. Drink 8 glasses of water
3. List 5 things you can do better regarding fitness

DAY 23 NOTES

DAY TWENTY-FOUR

"Fitness is like marriage. You can't cheat on it and expect it to work." – Bonnie Pfiester

MEDITATION~ Today, I abandon my old habits and take up new, more positive ones.

SUGGESTED VIDEO~ https://youtu.be/gvHPD7Y4N_0

How many times have you heard or read that you can't cheat the grind. It knows how hard you are working and the results will show to the world? This saying is prevalent in this book and on various social media outlets, because it's so true. You get what you give in all things. "It takes 4 weeks for you to see your body changing; it takes 8 weeks for your friends and family; it takes 12 weeks for the rest of the world." I don't know who initially made this quote, but I know for a fact that it's true. Keep going. Keep striving. Keep making yourself a priority. The daily fitness grind will broadcast your hard work to the world in no time! The twenty-fourth day of badassery assignment is as follows;

1. 15 to 30 minutes of exercise
2. Drink 8 glasses of water
3. List 5 distinct promises to meet or exceed your goals

DAY 24 NOTES

45 Days to Badass   BGP   *Julia Press Simmons*

DAY TWENTY-FIVE

"The only bad workout is the one that didn't happen." unknown

MEDITATION~ I love being physically fit and I lose enough weight so that I am at my ideal weight.

SUGGESTED VIDEO~ https://youtu.be/3wyp1Uqt34A

Scheduling regular rest intervals into your fitness routine is vitally important to your overall health, but slacking off for shits and giggles should never be an option. It is so easy to slip back into old habits especially when you are just starting to make better choices concerning your wellbeing. I know that, at any given moment, life can throw you a mean ass curveball. Things can get real bad and real busy, however, you have to remember that working out is something that you do for you. Always make your health and fitness a priority. Never quit on you. Push past the lazy. Push past the tendency to procrastinate. Push past any and all negative thoughts and feelings. Remember your value, and treat yourself accordingly. The twenty-fifth day of badassery assignment is as follows;

1. 15 to 30 minutes of exercise
2. Drink 8 glasses of water
3. List 3 of your major excuses and 3 ways to eliminate them.

56

DAY 25 NOTES

DAY TWENTY-SIX

"First you feel like dying, then you feel reborn."
unknown

MEDITATION~ Every day in every way I am approaching my ideal weight.

SUGGESTED VIDEO~ https://youtu.be/m-N18WuhCRQ

Get comfortable with being uncomfortable. Learn to love the aches and pains because they are proof positive that you are working your ass off. I sometimes have days where I dread working out. I stare at the TV screen with an attitude for a good fifteen or twenty minutes before I finally press play on my DVD remote. I can spend a whole half hour in the gym's parking lot giving myself a good talking to. I need the pep talk. I am human and I often struggle on my weight loss journey just like everyone else. Changing your life can is hard as hell, and waking up early to workout can be a major pain in the ass. But, Baby, when it's over, and I gave it all I got, I feel like a champion. All I want is for you to feel that way too. The twenty-sixth day of badassery assignment is as follows;

1. 15 to 30 minutes of exercise
2. Drink 8 glasses of water
3. List the positive emotions and rewards from sticking to your workout routine

DAY 26 NOTES

DAY TWENTY-SEVEN

"*We are what we repeatedly do. Excellence, therefore, is not an act but a habit.*" – Aristotle

MEDITATION~ I act with confidence having a general plan and accept plans are open to alteration

SUGGESTED VIDEO~
https://youtu.be/FXAcsxn0pQM

No one walks in the gym for the first time, and smashes a Mr. Olympia workout. You won't start out lifting heavy or running a 10k on the treadmill or elliptical trainer. It doesn't work that way. You have to build up to it. If you can only do ten minutes on the elliptical or stationary bike, then do ten minutes, but do the hell out of them. Day by day, workout by workout, you will get stronger. You will run faster, and be able to lift heavier without hurting yourself. The secret to excellence is in the small things. Excellence is hidden inside of daily commitment. Your will is strengthened with repetition. The twenty-seventh day of badassery assignment is as follows;

1. 15 to 30 minutes of exercise
2. Drink 8 glasses of water
3. Compare your workout times and endurance from week one until now, and then rejoice in your progress

DAY 27 NOTES

DAY TWENTY-EIGHT

"Stamina, speed, strength, skill and spirit. But the greatest of these is spirit." – **Ken Doherty**

MEDITATION~ I will focus on building my inner strength

SUGGESTED VIDEO~ https://youtu.be/qwlsF17GGYl

One of my favorite quotes of all time is Mark Twain's "It's not the size of the dog in the fight; it's the size of the fight in the dog." How big is the fight inside of you? How strong is your spirit??? These two questions will determine whether you win lose or draw on your journey to health and wellness. You can have a membership to the finest gym with state of the art equipment; you can have the latest fitness DVD, and buy a million books like this one, but if you don't strengthen your resolve, feed your spirit, and consistently flex your willpower muscle you will lose. It's a hard truth. Almost everything works if you work it, and nothing will work unless you do the inner work that your spirit requires. The twenty-eighth day of badassery assignment is as follows;

1. 15 to 30 minutes of exercise
2. Drink 8 glasses of water
3. List 5 relaxing activities that nourish your peace of mind, and incorporate them throughout your week

DAY 28 NOTES

DAY TWENTY-NINE

"We do not stop exercising because we grow old – we grow old because we stop exercising." ~ Dr. Kenneth Cooper

MEDITATION~ life is beautiful and I enjoy life by staying fit and maintaining my ideal weight.
SUGGESTED VIDEO~ https://youtu.be/Q23Exmnio8s

You want to take a sip from the fountain of youth? Well get up off your ass and move that thing all around. Daily exercise is scientifically proven to add years to your life, and shave years off of your appearance. According to the good people at Harvard and Brigham and Women's Hospital and the National Cancer Institute's study, 75 minutes of brisk walking per week equates to an extra 1.8 years of life expectancy as opposed to staying sedentary. Increase that to 150–299 minutes of brisk walking per week and the gain in life expectancy goes up to 3.4 years. Make it 450 minutes per week and the estimated life expectancy jumps by 4.5 years. You don't just feel better, you look better and that's just awesome. The twenty-ninth day of badassery assignment is as follows;

1. 15 to 30 minutes of exercise
2. Drink 8 glasses of water
3. List the changes to your appearance, note how far you have come

DAY 29 NOTES

DAY THIRTY

"You've got what it takes but it takes everything you've got." unknown

MEDITATION~ I choose to stay on track.

SUGGESTED VIDEO~ **https://youtu.be/jcVK_5nGOcM**

I would bet good money that you are a great parent, a good sibling; employee, neighbor, and you're probably someone's best friend. That is awesome. You're an amazing person, but how good are you to you? I want you to make yourself a priority and do so every day. I want you to pray for yourself, meditate for your peace of mind, and give your fitness routine all that you've got. Putting your wellbeing first should become second nature to you, and it's not selfish, it's necessary. You cannot continually give to others without giving to yourself. This is the quickest way to run your well dry. At the end of the day, caring for yourself is one of the best ways to care for your loved ones. The thirtieth day of badassery assignment is as follows;

1. 15 to 30 minutes of exercise
2. Drink 8 glasses of water
3. List 5 things you can start doing for you daily that you wouldn't hesitate to do for a loved one

DAY 30 NOTES

DAY THIRTY-ONE

"If you always put limits on everything you do, physical or anything else. It will spread into your work and into your life. There are no limits. There are only plateaus, and you must not stay there, you must go beyond them."
– Bruce Lee

MEDITATION~ I boldly go in the direction of my dreams

SUGGESTED VIDEO~ https://youtu.be/ZXTMGApEYHw

I used to put limits on all of my fitness efforts. I thought I could never do a burpee. I can't do pushups. I can't hold a plank for a minute. I can't lift that, I can't do this. These thoughts were ongoing. It kept me from reaching my potential. I convinced myself that all I could actually do was walk on a treadmill and put in 5 to 10 minutes on an elliptical trainer. I no longer do that. I no longer place limitations on anything I attempt to do in life. Instead, I ask how. How can I sustain a plank? How can I master a burpee? I erased can't and started to really try. You can accomplish anything if you open yourself up to the possibilities. Change the way you think about yourself and your potential, and you change your world. The thirty-first day of badassery assignment is as follows;

1. 15 to 30 minutes of exercise
2. Drink 8 glasses of water
3. List 3 things you think you can't do physically and then pledge to work on them 3 days a week

DAY 31 NOTES

DAY THIRTY-TWO

***"Pain is temporary. Quitting lasts forever."* – Lance Armstrong**

MEDITATION~ I face all obstacles with great courage and tenacity.

SUGGESTED VIDEO~ https://youtu.be/IzbCLooj-M8

The first time that I walked seven miles was on Kelly's Drive. I had an overwhelming urge to push myself. I remember walking down the river 3.5 miles before I turned around to head back. I was about a half a mile away from my car when my body started to hurt mercilessly. I started to cry. I thought that I wasn't going to make it back to my car. I was going to have to call someone to pick me up and drive me back. I couldn't go on. Then people who were walking along the trail started clapping for me and cheering me on. They shouted, "You can do it. You can do it. Keep going! Your mind wants to quit, but your body is capable." I took one painful step after the other, and made it to my car. The stranger aka angels all clapped for me, and hugged me. That was the most beautiful thing I experienced on my weight loss journey thus far. That was the day that I learned pain was temporary, quitting last forever. The thirty-second day of badassery assignment is as follows;

1. 15 to 30 minutes of exercise
2. Drink 8 glasses of water
3. List 3 ways to push yourself this week

DAY 32 NOTES

DAY THIRTY-THREE

"Success seems to be connected with action. Successful people keep moving. They make mistakes, but they don't quit." – **Conrad Hilton**

MEDITATION~ I face and conquer my fears with swift, decisive action.

SUGGESTED VIDEO~ https://youtu.be/LsstKVAWPTc

A note on bad days... THEY HAPPEN! Sometimes bad days are few and far between, and sometimes they are relentless and come at you back to back. They are a fact of life and you don't have to be on a weight loss journey to experience them. As sure as the Earth will spin on its Axis, and the sun will rise and set, you will have a bad day. Life will stress you out. Heartache will spread from your chest down to your toes. Your own personal rain cloud will park itself right above your head. You can't escape bad days, but you can learn to power through them. Action is your secret weapon. Nothing can kick a bad day in the teeth more than being productive, and carrying on. I use to mope through my hard days. I would throw myself a pity party, and invite anyone and everyone who would listen to my blues. Not anymore. I now know that action and hard work is not only the keys to success, it is also the antidote for bad days. The thirty-third day of badassery assignment is as follows;

1. 15 to 30 minutes of exercise
2. Drink 8 glasses of water
3. List 5 positive things to do on a bad day

DAY 33 NOTES

DAY THIRTY-FOUR

"Just don't give up trying to do what you really want to do. Where there is love and inspiration, I don't think you can go wrong." – Ella Fitzgerald

MEDITATION~ I will remain confident and unaffected by negative attitudes around me
SUGGESTED VIDEO~ https://youtu.be/aQBc-X21Gbg

Every now and again I have to go through old pictures and take in the look I had when I weighed over 300 pounds. I would do this whenever I get discouraged about slow progress or no progress, and I would do this whenever I felt my goals were just too far out of my reach. Going through those pictures worked like a charm. I realize that I may not be where I want to be, but I am nowhere near the starting line. I stare at the woman in those pictures, and marvel at how much I have changed. I'm not her anymore. She didn't love herself. She was depressed, anxious, and never really sure about anything. She was weak, but I am not. Seeing those pictures is proof positive of how strong I have become. Wonder Woman, a shero fully capable of saving the damn day. The thirty-fourth day of badassery assignment is as follows;

1. 15 to 30 minutes of exercise
2. Drink 8 glasses of water
3. List 5 major changes in your appearance since you started on your journey, and then celebrate

DAY 34 NOTES

DAY THIRTY-FIVE

"You're not obligated to win. You're obligated to keep trying. Do the best you can do every day." – Jason Mraz

MEDITATION~ I trust and believe in myself, and I let go of the negative.

SUGGESTED VIDEO~ https://youtu.be/754f1w90gQU

You will not lose ten, twenty, thirty, or fifty pounds today. You will not be able to climb a mountain today or lap an ocean. No one is looking at you and expecting miracles. You are not required to bring home the gold in an Olympic competition; all you are required to do is your best, whatever your best may be. Ask yourself how many times have you gone above and beyond for someone else. How many times have you placed someone else's needs before your own? You are a champion who is used to going the distance for everyone but yourself. That has to stop you are a priority and you deserve your best effort. Give yourself a chance. Do the absolute best for you, and before long you will end up exactly where you need to be. Remember you are not required to win; you're just required to give it all you got! The thirty-fifth day of badassery assignment is as follows;

1. 15 to 30 minutes of exercise
2. Drink 8 glasses of water
3. List 5 ways to try harder, recommit to your fitness

DAY 35 NOTES

DAY THIRTY-SIX

"The body achieves what the mind believes."
unknown

MEDITATION~ I can do this, I am doing this, my body is losing weight right now.

SUGGESTED VIDEO~ https://youtu.be/QS2vv72R2Xl

Today we will revisit visualization because it's one of the most powerful tools in your arsenal. "If you can see it, you most definitely can achieve it." That quote may seem cliché, however, quotes become cliché from overuse, and if everyone is using it there has to be something to it. So, do me a favor, after you finish reading this, and before you begin your action plan, close your eyes and visualize the body you want. Visualize your goal weight and ideal measurements. Once the image is clear, commit your vision to memory, and keep it in the forefront of your mind today. Every exercise you do today, every morsel of food you put in your mouth, and everything you tell yourself should be in honor of that vision. It might seem silly at first, but I am writing from experience, and trust me it works. Close your eyes and envision the best you possible! The thirty-sixth day of badassery assignment is as follows;

1. 15 to 30 minutes of exercise
2. Drink 8 glasses of water
3. List 5 fitness goals and 5 personal dreams

DAY 36 NOTES

DAY THIRTY-SEVEN

"I'm not telling you it is going to be easy, I'm telling you it is going to be worth it."

MEDITATION~ Each day I believe in myself more and more

SUGGESTED VIDEO~ https://youtu.be/sWbABaYr-k8

No one seems to talk about how hard this journey is, and that's a shame. I believe with all my heart that if people knew exactly how hard changing your lifestyle is more people would be better equipped to handle it. It's not easy at all, it's rather hard, but being overweight is hard, being sick is hard, and maintaining a healthy lifestyle is hard. You just have to choose your hard! We are on day 37 of 45 Days to Badass, and if you stuck it out with me this far, I know that you are tough enough to make your dreams a reality. Getting out of shape doesn't happen overnight, and getting into shape is a lifelong commitment. It's not an easy process, but it's necessary and you are worth it! The thirty-seventh day of badassery assignment is as follows;

1. 15 to 30 minutes of exercise
2. Drink 8 glasses of water
3. List 3 hard things about your fitness journey, and 3 ways to push past it

DAY 37 NOTES

DAY THIRTY-EIGHT

"Toughness is in the soul and spirit, not in the muscles." **unknown**

MEDITATION~ I am guided in my every step by Spirit who leads me towards what I must know and do.

SUGGESTED VIDEO~ https://youtu.be/7dg1rCq0ulQ

Did you know that the average body has almost no limitations? Most people are as capable of completing a triathlon as an Olympic athlete. The difference is in the training, strength of will, and mental aptitude. Your spirit will determine how far you go on this journey, so it is very important that you nourish it and feed it along the way. As we discussed yesterday, this journey is hard, and you will need to flex your will in order to win. I didn't start seeing progress until I incorporated prayer, meditation, and inspiration into my daily routine. My process was incomplete and feeding my spirit rounded it out, it added the balance that I desperately needed. I started feeling better, happier, and more at peace. The more I nurtured my soul, the more I realized that limitations are illusions. The thirty-eighth day of badassery assignment is as follows;

1. 15 to 30 minutes of exercise
2. Drink 8 glasses of water
3. List 5 ways prayer has impacted your life

DAY 38 NOTES

DAY THIRTY-NINE

Exercise to stimulate, not to annihilate. The world wasn't formed in a day, and neither were we. Set small goals and build upon them. ~ Lee Haney

MEDITATION~ I am transforming into someone who is happy and positive
SUGGESTED VIDEO~ https://youtu.be/5pCMbm6xWM0

Slow and steady wins the race. You will be surprised at the difference small consistent changes can make over a long period of time. I started my journey by walking to the corner store. After a few days I made it around the block. I took baby steps, and was very kind to myself during the process. .
In the past my self-esteem was very low, so loving myself and taking care of my self was a new concept. Physical fitness is a beautiful way to take care of your body. Make it a positive experience and love yourself every step of the way. The thirty-ninth day of badassery assignment is as follows;

1. 15 to 30 minutes of exercise
2. Drink 8 glasses of water
3. List 5 things you love about yourself

DAY 39 NOTES

DAY FORTY

"Practice doesn't make perfect, it makes permanent." Dr. Eric Thomas

MEDITATION~ I am confident that I can achieve anything

SUGGESTED VIDEO~ https://youtu.be/mX5oEIb5u9E

I used to have a dieter's mindset. I knew that eating right and working out would get me to my goal weight, but I would always limit those actions to a specific time frame. As soon as I made any significant progress I would revert back to my old habits and balloon up to my previous weight. That is the yo-yo effect. I now know that this is a lifelong commitment. It takes anywhere from three weeks to two and a half months to form a habit, so I designed this book to land in between those time frames. How many times have you heard the phrase "We are what we repeatedly do?" We are creatures of habit, however, we have the power to choose positive actions and make positive decisions. The fortieth day of badassery assignment is as follows;

1. 15 to 30 minutes of exercise
2. Drink 8 glasses of water
3. List 2 bad habits to break, and 2 good habits to start

DAY 40 NOTES

DAY FORTY-ONE

It's not about weight, it's about fitness, and one component of being fit is to have relatively low body fat, because fat is not very efficient, whereas muscle is.

Deborah Bull

MEDITATION~ I am a person who easily accepts new challenges.

SUGGESTED VIDEO~ https://youtu.be/6x47lkgljwA

After about three months of walking I knew I needed more. I joined Planet Fitness and fell in love with the Elliptical machine. I loved to covered in sweat (it made me feel like I was doing something), and after forty-five minutes to an hour on the Elliptical Trainer I was soaking wet. I was losing weight steadily, but my body wasn't changing. I talked to a trainer at the gym who said I needed to start lifting weights, and or start resistance training. That's when I purchased Shaun T's Hip-Hop abs and T25 program. The change to my body was amazing. The numbers on the scale stopped moving down which was distressing until the trainer at the gym told me that I was building muscle. I now lift weights three days a week. The forty-first day of badassery assignment is as follows;

1. 15 to 30 minutes of exercise
2. Drink 8 glasses of water
3. List and research a couple of resistance programs and incorporate them into your workout

DAY 41 NOTES

DAY FORTY-TWO

Exercise is done against one's wishes and maintained only because the alternative is worse. ~ George A. Sheehan

MEDITATION~ I feel excitement when life brings challenges to me, and I gladly accept them without any guilt or anxiety.

SUGGESTED VIDEO~ https://youtu.be/_zBZcZWNxAc

All the benefits you gain from working out are reversed when you stop or don't start exercising. You will find every single pound that you lost. You become vulnerable to a wide range of diseases including Diabetes and Hypertension. Your energy level decreases. You lose bone density and your muscles start wasting away, and that is just the tip of the iceberg. There are a host of mental and emotional draw backs from neglecting to exercise. I don't work out because I hate my body. I work out because I love it. I love myself, and I want the best for myself mentally, emotionally, and physically. The forty-second day of badassery assignment is as follows;

1. 15 to 30 minutes of exercise
2. Drink 8 glasses of water
3. List 5 things that can happen or has happened to you when you don't exercise

DAY 42 NOTES

DAY FORTY-THREE

I think exercise tests us in so many ways, our skills, our hearts, and our ability to bounce back after setbacks. This is the inner beauty of sports and competition, and it can serve us all well as adult athletes. ~Peggy Fleming

MEDITATION~ I feel my desire for fat-rich foods dissolving.

SUGGESTED VIDEO~ https://youtu.be/FvCozyHkm5E

The greatest war a person will wage in their lifetime is the battle within. Once you conquer yourself you can overcome any and everything. That is the core mission of becoming the best version of you. Along the way you learn that you are your only competition. You are your problem, but you are also your solution. No one can force you to get up early to workout, or go to the gym after a long day at work. No one can make you make healthier food choices. It's all you, baby. Every time you make the best decisions for yourself you defeat your lower desires. You become stronger, healthier and closer to your goals! The forty-third day of badassery assignment is as follows;

1. 15 to 30 minutes of exercise
2. Drink 8 glasses of water
3. List 5 things that you have conquered along the way.

DAY 43 NOTES

DAY FORTY-FOUR

"I hated every minute of training, but I said, 'Don't quit. Suffer now and live the rest of your life as a champion.'" ~ Muhammad Ali

MEDITATION~ My ability to conquer my challenges is limitless; my potential to succeed is infinite.

SUGGESTED VIDEO~ https://youtu.be/H1sXTmaqRHU

It's day 44 and you are a champion. You made it to the finish line. You have decided to love yourself and make yourself a priority. Congratulations. I would like to tell you that it gets easier from here on out, but I don't lie about important shit. It will still be hard. You still have to fight to be fit, but there is an upside. You now know exactly what you are capable of. You know that you can make a commitment to yourself, and you have the inner strength to honor it. You know that feeding your spirit and having faith in the process is one of the most important aspects of your journey. You got this. You got it in the bag! The forty-fourth day of badassery assignment is as follows;

1. 15 to 30 minutes of exercise
2. Drink 8 glasses of water
3. List 5 things you are going to take away from this book

DAY 44 NOTES

DAY FORTY-FIVE

**The finish line is just the beginning of a whole new race.
-Unknown**

MEDITATION~ Today, I abandon my old habits and take up new, more positive ones.

SUGGESTED VIDEO~ https://youtu.be/350F0VsECvo

Wooo hooo! You have arrived at the last day, and you are now a badass. Allow yourself a moment of reflection and then rush full speed ahead into the next chapter of your fitness life. Join the gym. Hire a personal trainer, stream Daily Burn, or my personal favorite Beach Body. You have proven that you can do this. You have the testicular fortitude to accomplish any and everything that you put your mind to. The forty-fifth day of badassery assignment is as follows;

1. 15 to 30 minutes of exercise
2. Drink 8 glasses of water
3. Research the next leg of your fitness journey, and jump right into it. Don't take a break. It's not time to relax, it's time to move forward, and I am so very proud of you!

DAY 45 NOTES

Positive Affirmation Reference

http://www.freeaffirmations.org/self-esteem-positive-affirmations\

http://enlightenmentportal.com/affirmations/positive-affirmations-for-weight-loss-and-confidence/

http://bmindful.com/affirmations/strength

http://www.more-selfesteem.com/affirmations.htm

http://www.self-help-and-self-development.com/weight-loss-affirmations.html

Weight loss and fitness books
By Julia Press Simmons

Fuck it, I'm Fat: My Weight Loss Journey

Oh Shit, I lost Some Weight: 60 lbs in 6 Months

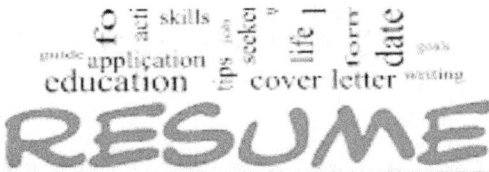

Paradigm Shift Resume Service
Do you need a resume? Let me help
you get the career you deserve.
Send me an old copy, No old copy?
No problem! Make the Shift, the
Paradigm Shift and get into the world
of work.
We also provide cover letters,
professional reference letters and
much more. Contact us today:
pshiftresume@gmail.com or Call:
215.225.0695

Send the following:
Name, Address, Email
Phone Number, School Information
Your current and previous jobs
The positions you held, and the years
you held them. What time of positions
you are seeking
And watch us work magic!

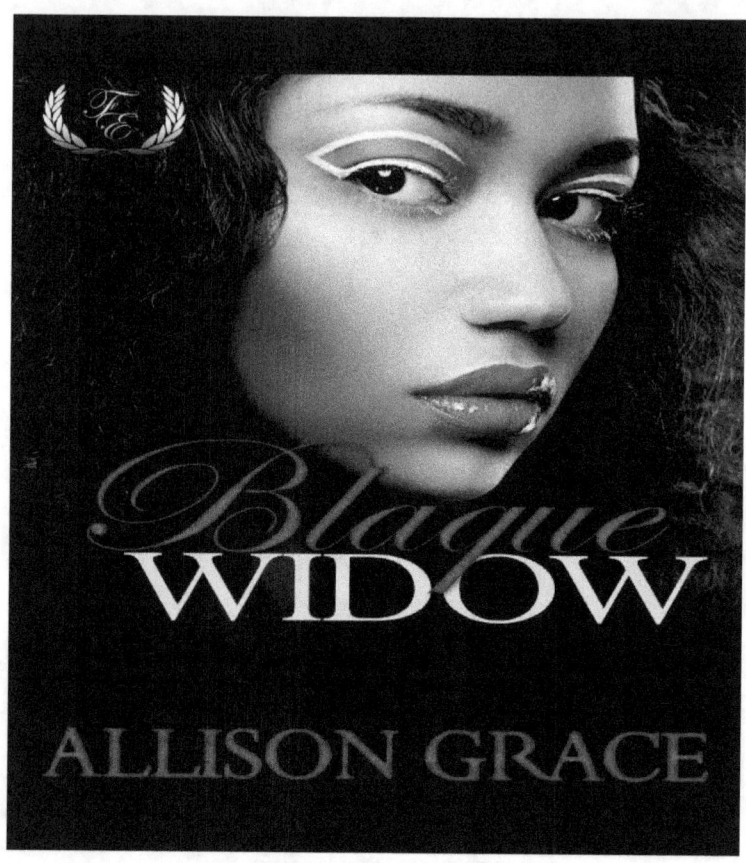

Are you ready to indulge in the sleeper hit of 2015? Meet Taryn Durand. She loves love, but it doesn't love her back. She experienced heartache in the worst way yet with a smile on her face still seeks out her happily ever after. Suddenly, her "Prince Charming" turns into something so wicked, she can only escape it by destroying it. See what secrets unfold and how reality bites as you enter Taryn's world...

www.ingramcontent.com/pod-product-compliance
Lightning Source LLC
Chambersburg PA
CBHW062041280526
45788CB00003B/1072